Holistic Wellness: Achieving Optimal Health and Balance in the Modern World

Brenda J. Smith

Table of contents

III. Nourishing Your Body for Optimal Health

A. The role of nutrition in holistic wellness

B. Understanding macronutrients, micronutrients, and their sources

C. Exploring mindful eating and intuitive eating practices

D. Addressing common dietary challenges and promoting a balanced diet

IV. Movement and Physical Fitness for a Balanced Life

A. The benefits of regular physical activity for holistic wellness

B. Exploring different types of exercise and their specific benefits

C. Designing a personalized fitness plan based on individual goals and preferences

D. Integrating movement into daily routines and combating sedentary lifestyles

V. Nurturing Mental and Emotional Well-Being

A. Understanding the mind-body connection and its impact on holistic wellness

B. Techniques for managing stress, anxiety, and negative emotions

C. Cultivating resilience and fostering positive mental health habits

D. Exploring mindfulness, meditation, and relaxation techniques

VI. Creating a Healthy and Supportive Environment

A. The impact of the physical environment on well-being

B. Promoting a clutter-free and organized space for mental clarity

C. Enhancing sleep quality through optimal bedroom design and sleep hygiene practices

D.   Building   supportive   relationships   and
fostering social connections

VII. Holistic Wellness in the Digital Age
A. Navigating the challenges and opportunities
of technology in holistic wellness
B. Mindful use of digital devices and managing
screen time
C. Utilizing digital resources and apps for
holistic wellness support
D.   Striking   a   balance   between   digital
engagement and real-life connections

VIII. Integrating Holistic Wellness Practices into Daily Life
A. Developing sustainable habits and routines
for long-term well-being
B.   Overcoming   barriers   and   maintaining
motivation on the wellness journey
C. Strategies for self-reflection, goal-setting, and
tracking progress

D. Celebrating milestones and embracing the ongoing process of holistic wellness

IX. Holistic Wellness for a Sustainable Future
A. Exploring the connection between holistic wellness and environmental consciousness
B. Promoting eco-friendly practices for a healthier planet and personal well-being
C. Advocating for holistic wellness in communities and society at large

X. Conclusion
A. Reflecting on the transformative power of holistic wellness
B. Inspiring readers to embrace a balanced and fulfilling life in the modern world
C. Encouraging ongoing exploration and self-discovery on the path to optimal health and well-being

Chapter 1:

Introduction:

In an era defined by constant connectivity, information overload, and a never-ending quest for balance, the pursuit of holistic wellness has gained significant importance. Welcome to "Holistic Wellness: Achieving Optimal Health and Balance in the Modern World," an eBook dedicated to exploring the profound impact of holistic wellness in our lives today. In this transformative journey, we will delve into the core concepts of holistic wellness, beginning with its definition and its deep interconnectedness with our physical, mental, and emotional well-being.

A. Defining Holistic Wellness and Its Significance in the Modern World

In this opening chapter, we lay the foundation for our exploration by defining holistic wellness and its immense significance in the modern world. Holistic wellness encompasses an all-encompassing approach to health and well-being, recognizing that true vitality and balance go beyond mere absence of illness. We delve into the idea of treating the whole person, addressing not just the physical body, but also the mind and emotions. By understanding the essence of holistic wellness, we unlock the potential for a more vibrant, fulfilling, and balanced life.

B. Exploring the Interconnectedness of Physical, Mental, and Emotional Well-Being

In this chapter, we embark on a journey to uncover the intricate interconnectedness of our physical, mental, and emotional well-being. We explore how each aspect influences and impacts the others, recognizing that they are not isolated entities but interconnected facets of our holistic self. By understanding and embracing this interconnectedness, we gain insights into the profound ways in which our physical health, mental clarity, and emotional resilience are intertwined. This understanding becomes the cornerstone of achieving optimal health and balance in the modern world.

As we navigate the remaining chapters of this eBook, we will delve deeper into various aspects of holistic wellness, providing practical guidance, evidence-based strategies, and actionable steps to support your journey toward a more balanced and vibrant life.

Chapter 2:

Understanding the Foundations of Holistic Wellness

In our quest for holistic wellness, it is essential to understand the foundational elements that shape our overall well-being. In this chapter, we will explore the key components of holistic wellness, recognize the profound impact of lifestyle choices on our health, and emphasize the importance of prevention and proactive self-care.

Exploring the Key Components of Holistic Wellness

Holistic wellness encompasses a holistic approach to health and balance that extends beyond just physical well-being. We will delve into the various dimensions of holistic wellness, including physical, mental, emotional, and spiritual aspects. By recognizing the

11

interconnected nature of these dimensions, we gain a comprehensive understanding of the multiple facets that contribute to our overall well-being.

Recognizing the Impact of Lifestyle Choices on Overall Health

Our lifestyle choices play a pivotal role in shaping our health and well-being. We will explore the impact of factors such as nutrition, physical activity, sleep, stress management, and environmental influences on our overall wellness. By understanding the significance of these lifestyle choices, we can make informed decisions and create positive habits that support our journey towards optimal health and balance.

Emphasizing the Importance of Prevention and Proactive Self-Care

Prevention and proactive self-care are fundamental principles of holistic wellness. We will discuss the importance of taking a proactive approach to our well-being by adopting preventive measures and engaging in self-care practices. By prioritizing prevention, we can minimize the risk of illness, enhance our overall vitality, and maintain long-term well-being. We will also explore practical strategies and techniques to incorporate proactive self-care into our daily lives, nurturing our physical, mental, and emotional well-being.

Throughout this chapter, we will provide insights, research-based information, and practical tips to help you understand the foundations of holistic wellness. By gaining a deeper understanding of the key components of holistic wellness, recognizing the impact of lifestyle choices on our overall health, and embracing prevention and proactive self-care, you will be empowered to take control of your well-being and embark on a transformative journey towards optimal health and balance in the modern world.

As we continue our exploration in the subsequent chapters, we will delve deeper into specific aspects of holistic wellness, offering guidance, tools, and practices to support your ongoing journey towards achieving holistic well-being in the modern world.

Chapter 3:

Nourishing Your Body for Optimal Health

A vital aspect of holistic wellness is nourishing our bodies with proper nutrition. In this chapter, we will explore the role of nutrition in holistic wellness, understand the importance of macronutrients and micronutrients, delve into mindful eating and intuitive eating practices, and address common dietary challenges while promoting a balanced diet.

The Role of Nutrition in Holistic Wellness

Nutrition forms the foundation of our well-being. We will examine how the food we consume affects our physical, mental, and emotional health. By understanding the essential role of nutrition in supporting our body's functions, we can make informed choices that align with our holistic wellness goals.

Understanding Macronutrients, Micronutrients, and Their Sources

To nourish our bodies effectively, it is crucial to comprehend macronutrients (carbohydrates, proteins, and fats) and micronutrients (vitamins and minerals) and their sources. We will explore the specific roles these nutrients play in our overall health and well-being, helping us create a balanced and nutrient-rich diet.

Exploring Mindful Eating and Intuitive Eating Practices

Mindful eating and intuitive eating practices empower us to develop a healthy relationship with food and our bodies. We will delve into the principles of mindful eating, emphasizing the importance of being present and aware during meals. Additionally, we will explore intuitive eating, which involves listening to our body's cues and honoring our hunger and fullness signals. By embracing these practices, we can foster a harmonious connection with food and cultivate a sustainable approach to nourishing our bodies.

Addressing Common Dietary Challenges and Promoting a Balanced Diet

Many individuals face dietary challenges due to various factors such as allergies, dietary restrictions, or conflicting information. We will address these common challenges and provide strategies to overcome them. Additionally, we will emphasize the significance of a balanced diet that incorporates a variety of whole foods, encouraging moderation and mindfulness in our dietary choices.

By exploring these topics, you will gain a deeper understanding of the role of nutrition in holistic wellness. You will be equipped with the knowledge to make informed decisions about your dietary choices, embrace mindful and intuitive eating practices, and navigate common dietary challenges while maintaining a balanced and nourishing diet. Together, let us embark on a journey of nourishing our bodies for optimal health and well-being in the modern world.

Chapter 4:

Movement and Physical Fitness for a Balanced Life

Physical activity and regular exercise are essential components of holistic wellness. In this chapter, we will explore the benefits of regular physical activity, delve into different types of exercise and their specific benefits, guide you in designing a personalized fitness plan based on your goals and preferences, and provide strategies for integrating movement into your daily routines to combat sedentary lifestyles.

The Benefits of Regular Physical Activity for Holistic Wellness

Regular physical activity offers numerous benefits for our holistic well-being. We will explore how exercise positively impacts our physical health, mental clarity, emotional well-being, and overall quality of life. From increased cardiovascular health to improved mood and stress management, we will uncover the wide-ranging benefits that physical activity brings to our holistic wellness.

Exploring Different Types of Exercise and Their Specific Benefits

Exercise comes in various forms, and each offers unique benefits. We will explore different types of exercise, including aerobic exercises, strength training, flexibility exercises, and mind-body practices such as yoga or tai chi. By understanding the specific benefits of each type, you can choose exercises that align with your preferences and goals, ensuring a well-rounded approach to your fitness routine.

Designing a Personalized Fitness Plan Based on Individual Goals and Preferences

Designing a fitness plan that suits your individual goals and preferences is crucial for long-term adherence and success. We will guide you in identifying your fitness goals, considering factors such as endurance, strength, flexibility, and overall well-being. With this knowledge, you will be able to create a personalized fitness plan that is enjoyable, sustainable, and tailored to your specific needs.

Integrating Movement into Daily Routines and Combating Sedentary Lifestyles

In today's sedentary world, it is vital to find ways to incorporate movement into our daily lives. We will explore practical strategies for integrating physical activity into your daily routines, whether at home, work, or during leisure time. From incorporating walking breaks to incorporating active hobbies, we will provide actionable tips to help you combat sedentary lifestyles and embrace a more active and balanced approach to daily living.

By exploring the benefits of regular physical activity, understanding different types of exercise and their specific benefits, designing a personalized fitness plan, and finding ways to integrate movement into your daily routines, you will be well-equipped to embrace a physically active lifestyle that enhances your holistic wellness. Together, let us embark on a journey of movement and physical fitness, nurturing our bodies and achieving optimal health and balance in the modern world.

Chapter 5:

Nurturing Mental and Emotional Well-Being

In our pursuit of holistic wellness, it is crucial to prioritize the nurturing of our mental and emotional well-being. In this chapter, we will explore the profound impact of the mind-body connection on holistic wellness, provide techniques for managing stress, anxiety, and negative emotions, guide you in cultivating resilience and fostering positive mental health habits, and introduce mindfulness, meditation, and relaxation techniques to support your mental and emotional well-being.

Understanding the Mind-Body Connection and Its Impact on Holistic Wellness

The mind and body are intricately connected, and understanding this connection is vital for achieving optimal holistic wellness. We will delve into the science behind the mind-body connection, exploring how our thoughts, emotions, and beliefs can influence our physical health and well-being. By recognizing the profound impact of the mind-body connection, we can harness its power to support our holistic wellness journey.

Techniques for Managing Stress, Anxiety, and Negative Emotions

Stress, anxiety, and negative emotions can significantly impact our mental and emotional well-being. We will provide practical techniques and strategies to manage these challenges effectively. From stress reduction exercises and relaxation techniques to cognitive-behavioral approaches and emotional regulation practices, you will learn valuable tools to navigate and mitigate the impact of stress, anxiety, and negative emotions on your holistic wellness.

Cultivating Resilience and Fostering Positive Mental Health Habits

Building resilience and fostering positive mental health habits are essential for maintaining balance and well-being in the face of life's challenges. We will explore techniques to cultivate resilience, such as reframing perspectives, practicing self-compassion, and nurturing supportive relationships. Additionally, we will guide you in developing positive mental health habits, including self-care routines, gratitude practices, and the power of positive affirmations.

Exploring Mindfulness, Meditation, and Relaxation Techniques

Mindfulness, meditation, and relaxation techniques are powerful tools for nurturing mental and emotional well-being. We will introduce these practices, guiding you through mindfulness exercises, various meditation techniques, and relaxation strategies. By incorporating these techniques into your daily life, you can enhance self-awareness, promote inner calmness, and cultivate a deep sense of relaxation and balance.

By exploring the mind-body connection, learning techniques for managing stress and negative emotions, cultivating resilience, and embracing mindfulness, meditation, and relaxation practices, you will empower yourself to nurture your mental and emotional well-being on your holistic wellness journey. Together, let us embark on a path of self-care and self-discovery, fostering optimal mental and emotional health in the modern world.

Chapter 6:

Creating a Healthy and Supportive Environment

Our physical environment plays a significant role in our holistic wellness. In this chapter, we will explore the impact of the physical environment on our well-being, provide guidance on promoting a clutter-free and organized space for mental clarity, offer tips for enhancing sleep quality through optimal bedroom design and sleep hygiene practices, and emphasize the importance of building supportive relationships and fostering social connections for holistic wellness.

The Impact of the Physical Environment on Well-Being

Our surroundings can greatly influence our mental, emotional, and physical well-being. We will delve into the ways in which our physical environment affects us, from the colors and lighting in our living spaces to the natural elements present in our surroundings. By understanding this impact, we can make conscious choices to create an environment that nurtures our holistic wellness.

Promoting a Clutter-Free and Organized Space for Mental Clarity

Clutter and disorganization can hinder our mental clarity and contribute to feelings of stress and overwhelm. We will provide practical tips and strategies for decluttering and organizing our living and working spaces. By creating a clutter-free environment, we can promote a sense of calmness, focus, and mental clarity, allowing us to thrive in our daily lives.

Enhancing Sleep Quality through Optimal Bedroom Design and Sleep Hygiene Practices

Quality sleep is essential for our overall well-being. We will explore the impact of bedroom design on sleep quality, covering topics such as lighting, temperature, noise reduction, and comfortable bedding. Additionally, we will discuss sleep hygiene practices, including establishing a consistent sleep routine, creating a relaxing bedtime ritual, and minimizing electronic device usage before sleep. By optimizing our sleep environment and adopting healthy sleep habits, we can enhance the quality of our rest and rejuvenation.

Building Supportive Relationships and Fostering Social Connections

Human connection is vital for holistic wellness. We will emphasize the importance of building

30

and nurturing supportive relationships, both with ourselves and with others. We will explore strategies for cultivating meaningful connections, fostering open communication, and nurturing a supportive social network. By investing in relationships and fostering social connections, we can experience a sense of belonging, emotional support, and overall well-being.

By understanding the impact of the physical environment on well-being, promoting a clutter-free and organized space, enhancing sleep quality, and building supportive relationships and social connections, you will create a healthy and supportive environment that nurtures your holistic wellness. Together, let us create spaces that support our well-being and cultivate connections that enrich our lives in the modern world.

Chapter 7:

Holistic Wellness in the Digital Age

In today's digital age, technology has become an integral part of our lives, offering both opportunities and challenges in our pursuit of holistic wellness. In this chapter, we explore

32

how to navigate the digital landscape mindfully, harnessing its potential while avoiding its pitfalls. We delve into the following key aspects of holistic wellness in the digital age:

Navigating the Challenges and Opportunities of Technology in Holistic Wellness

The rapid advancement of technology brings a myriad of challenges and opportunities for our well-being. We discuss the potential negative impacts, such as excessive screen time, information overload, and the constant availability of distractions. At the same time, we uncover the positive aspects, such as access to health information, digital communities, and innovative tools that can support our holistic wellness journey.

Mindful Use of Digital Devices and Managing Screen Time

In this section, we emphasize the importance of mindfulness and intentionality when using digital devices. We explore strategies for managing screen time and establishing healthy boundaries to prevent digital overload and its associated negative effects on our well-being. By adopting mindful practices, we can develop a healthier relationship with technology and cultivate a more balanced and present lifestyle.

Utilizing Digital Resources and Apps for Holistic Wellness Support

The digital realm offers a wealth of resources and applications that can enhance our holistic wellness journey. We explore various digital tools, including fitness trackers, meditation apps, nutrition apps, and online communities, among others. We discuss how to effectively leverage these resources to support our physical, mental, and emotional well-being. By embracing technology consciously, we can tap into its potential to empower and guide us on our path to optimal health.

Striking a Balance Between Digital Engagement and Real-Life Connections

While technology enables us to connect with others globally, it is crucial to strike a balance between digital engagement and real-life connections. In this section, we delve into the importance of maintaining authentic, meaningful relationships and fostering genuine human connections. We explore strategies for finding harmony between our digital interactions and nurturing our social well-being offline. By prioritizing real-life connections, we can enrich our holistic wellness and cultivate a sense of belonging and support.

By navigating the challenges, embracing mindful practices, and utilizing digital resources wisely, we can harness the power of technology to support our holistic wellness journey. By striking a balance between digital engagement and real-life connections, we create a harmonious approach to well-being in the digital age. Together, let us embrace the opportunities technology presents while remaining grounded in our quest for optimal health and balance in the modern world.

Chapter 8:

Integrating Holistic Wellness Practices into Daily Life

In our pursuit of holistic wellness, it is essential to integrate wellness practices into our daily lives, ensuring long-term well-being and balance. In this chapter, we explore key strategies and techniques to help you seamlessly incorporate holistic wellness into your routine. We focus on the following four items:

Developing Sustainable Habits and Routines for Long-Term Well-Being

Creating sustainable habits is fundamental to achieving lasting results in our holistic wellness journey. We delve into the process of habit formation, emphasizing the importance of consistency and gradual progress. We discuss strategies for identifying and implementing sustainable practices, such as establishing a morning or evening routine, incorporating movement breaks throughout the day, and cultivating mindful eating habits. By developing sustainable habits, we create a solid foundation for our ongoing well-being.

Overcoming Barriers and Maintaining Motivation on the Wellness Journey

Throughout our holistic wellness journey, we may encounter obstacles and face moments of demotivation. In this section, we explore effective strategies for overcoming barriers and maintaining motivation. We discuss the power of mindset and self-compassion, offering techniques to overcome self-limiting beliefs and navigate through challenges. Additionally, we explore the importance of finding sources of inspiration, creating a supportive environment, and seeking accountability to stay motivated on our path to optimal health and balance.

Strategies for Self-Reflection, Goal-Setting, and Tracking Progress

Self-reflection and goal-setting are invaluable tools for our holistic wellness journey. We guide you through the process of self-reflection, helping you gain insight into your values, priorities, and areas for growth. We explore effective goal-setting techniques, ensuring that your goals align with your holistic wellness vision. Furthermore, we discuss the importance of tracking progress and celebrate small victories along the way. By incorporating these strategies, you can stay focused, measure your progress, and adjust your approach as needed.

Celebrating Milestones and Embracing the Ongoing Process of Holistic Wellness

Holistic wellness is not a destination; it is an ongoing process of growth and self-discovery. In this final item, we emphasize the significance of celebrating milestones and embracing the journey itself. We discuss the importance of self-care, self-compassion, and embracing the present moment. We encourage you to appreciate the progress you have made, no matter how small, and to find joy and fulfillment in the ongoing process of holistic wellness. By adopting this mindset, you can sustain your motivation and find deep satisfaction in your pursuit of optimal health and balance.

By integrating holistic wellness practices into your daily life, developing sustainable habits, overcoming barriers, and embracing self-reflection, you can create a transformative and fulfilling wellness journey. Remember to celebrate milestones, stay motivated, and appreciate the ongoing process of holistic wellness. Together, let us weave these practices into the fabric of our lives, unlocking the full potential of optimal health and balance in the modern world.

Chapter 9:

Holistic Wellness for a Sustainable Future

As we strive for holistic wellness, it is essential to recognize the profound connection between our well-being and the well-being of the planet. In this chapter, we explore the intersection of holistic wellness and environmental consciousness, promoting eco-friendly practices for a healthier planet and personal well-being. We focus on the following three items:

Exploring the Connection Between Holistic Wellness and Environmental Consciousness

We delve into the intrinsic link between holistic wellness and environmental consciousness, highlighting how our well-being is intimately tied to the health of the planet. We discuss the concept of "eco-wellness," which encompasses the belief that a sustainable and thriving environment is essential for our physical, mental, and emotional well-being. By recognizing this connection, we can cultivate a deeper appreciation for the Earth and work towards a more sustainable future.

Promoting Eco-Friendly Practices for a Healthier Planet and Personal Well-Being

In this section, we explore practical strategies for integrating eco-friendly practices into our daily lives. We discuss sustainable choices such as reducing waste, conserving energy and water, adopting a plant-based diet, supporting local and organic products, and embracing mindful consumption. These practices not only benefit the environment but also contribute to our personal well-being by fostering a sense of purpose, connection to nature, and a healthier lifestyle.

Advocating for Holistic Wellness in Communities and Society at Large

Creating a sustainable future requires collective action and advocacy. We discuss ways to promote holistic wellness in our communities and society at large. We explore the importance of education and awareness, empowering individuals to make informed choices and inspiring others to embrace a holistic approach to well-being. We also highlight the significance of collaboration, encouraging the formation of community initiatives, and supporting policies that prioritize holistic wellness and environmental sustainability.

By exploring the connection between holistic wellness and environmental consciousness, promoting eco-friendly practices, and advocating for holistic wellness in communities and society, we contribute to a sustainable future for both ourselves and the planet. Let us embrace the interconnectedness of our well-being and the well-being of the Earth, cultivating a harmonious relationship that nurtures both. Together, we can create a healthier and more sustainable world, where holistic wellness thrives for generations to come.

Chapter 10:

Conclusion

As we come to the end of this journey through "Holistic Wellness: Achieving Optimal Health and Balance in the Modern World," it is time to reflect on the transformative power of embracing a holistic approach to well-being. Throughout this eBook, we have explored the interconnectedness of our physical, mental, and emotional well-being, recognizing that true wellness encompasses all aspects of our lives. As we conclude, let us focus on three essential aspects:

Reflecting on the Transformative Power of Holistic Wellness

Through our exploration, we have witnessed the transformative power of holistic wellness. By embracing a comprehensive view of our well-being and integrating various practices, we can experience profound changes in our lives. We have learned that when we prioritize self-care, nourish our bodies with wholesome foods, engage in regular physical activity, nurture our mental and emotional well-being, and cultivate a supportive environment, we unlock our full potential for health and balance. Reflect on the progress you have made and the positive transformations you have experienced along your holistic wellness journey.

Inspiring Readers to Embrace a Balanced and Fulfilling Life in the Modern World

In today's fast-paced and interconnected world, finding balance and fulfillment can seem challenging. However, by embracing the principles of holistic wellness, we can navigate the complexities of modern life with grace and intention. I encourage you to take what you have learned and apply it to your daily life, seeking harmony in all areas. Embrace the power of mindfulness, self-compassion, and conscious choices as you create a life that aligns with your values and priorities. Remember that a balanced and fulfilling life is within your reach.

Encouraging Ongoing Exploration and Self-Discovery on the Path to Optimal Health and Well-Being

The journey to holistic wellness is not a destination but an ongoing process of self-discovery and growth. I encourage you to continue exploring and experimenting with different practices, adjusting them to fit your unique needs and preferences. Embrace curiosity, be open to new experiences, and remain committed to your well-being. Your path may evolve as you encounter new challenges and opportunities, but trust in your ability to navigate them with resilience and self-empowerment.

As we conclude this eBook, remember that holistic wellness is a lifelong journey that requires dedication, self-care, and conscious choices. Embrace the transformative power of holistic wellness, not just for your own well-being, but also for the well-being of the planet and the communities around you. By nurturing your physical, mental, and emotional health, you contribute to a harmonious and sustainable future. Embrace a balanced and fulfilling life, guided by the principles of holistic wellness, and inspire others to join you on this transformative path.

May you continue to explore, discover, and thrive on your journey towards optimal health and well-being. Embrace the interconnectedness of all aspects of your being, and may holistic wellness be your guide in creating a life of wholeness and balance in the modern world.

www.ingramcontent.com/pod-product-compliance
Lightning Source LLC
Chambersburg PA
CBHW070958260726
48661CB00007B/2745